A handbook of

Aortoarteritis
And
Ruptured Sinus
Of Valsalva

Alok Ranjan

Sr. Consultant – Cardiology
Care Hospitals
Surat

authorHOUSE®

AuthorHouse™
1663 Liberty Drive
Bloomington, IN 47403
www.authorhouse.com
Phone: 1 (800) 839-8640

Published by AuthorHouse 12/03/2015

ISBN: 978-1-5049-6309-1 (sc)
ISBN: 978-1-5049-6308-4 (hc)
ISBN: 978-1-5049-6307-7 (e)

Library of Congress Control Number: 2015919429

Print information available on the last page.

Dedication

Dedicated to my teachers (**Dr. (Mrs.) R. B. Amin, Dr. (Mrs.) S. S. Sirsikar and Dr. A. S. Mane**) and friends at Sassoon General Hospital and B J Medical college, Pune, Maharashtra, India

"One looks back with appreciation to the brilliant teachers, but with gratitude to those who touched our human feelings. The curriculum is so much necessary raw material, but warmth is the vital element for the growing plant and for the soul of the child.'

Carl Gustav Jung (1875-1961) Swiss psychologist and psychiatrist.

Index

Aortoarteritis (AA)

Definition

AA is a chronic inflammatory disease of unknown etiology that involves aorta and its major branches.
American College of Rheumatology (1990)

Modification suggested by Kinare et al
(Pathology and Radiology. Mumbai, Quest 1998; 69.)
AA is an idiopathic inflammatory disease of large elastic arteries occurring in the young and resulting in occlusive or ectatic changes mainly in aorta and its immediate branches as well as the pulmonary artery and its branches.

Synonyms
Takayasu arteritis (TA)
Reversed coarctation
"Pulseless" disease
Aortic arch syndrome
Occlusive thrombo-aortopathy: Coined by Ishikawa
    Describes the basic pathophysiology
Young female arteritis
Non-specific aortoarteritis

Etiology

Disease of **unknown etiology**

    Can be best described as "triggered by an external stimulus in genetically predisposed subjects"

Most favored theory is autoimmune inflammatory reaction

    Supported by increased levels of immunoglobulins
    Presence of anti aorta antibodies
        Not reported extensively by workers outside Japan
        Reported by Dhingra R, Talwar KK
    Presence of anti endothelial cell antibodies

Genetic studies

    Association with HLA system
    Kumar et al reported
        An increased frequency of HLA B5 and B21
        Decreased frequency of HLA B 35 and B 40

Linked to
        Rheumatic fever
            Proposed by Ask – Upmark
            Not valid now

Tuberculosis
    Reported by Japanese workers
    Supported by Kinare et al from India

Streptococcal infections
Rheumatoid arthritis
Other Collagen vascular disease

Pathophysiology

Histopathology:

Hallmark of the disease is a **granulomatous** lesion with giant cells.

Hence classified as '**giant cell arteritis**'

Phases of histopathological changes:

Active phase

Diffuse inflammation: Earliest phase
Starts at junction of media and adventitia
Spreads to adventitia and periadventitial tissues
Granuloma formation
Restricted to media, rarely seen in adventitia

Chronic phase

Adventitia is composed of collagen rich fibrous tissue
which may extend to periadventitial region
Adventitia becomes several times thicker than media
and becomes 'rigid pipe like' in appearance
Elastic fibers in media are replaced by scar tissue
Intima also becomes hyaline and several times thicker
than media

Healed phase

Appearances similar to chronic phase except inflammatory cells are scarce or absent

Pathological changes in Aorta

Shows one of the following changes
Localized involvement
2 – 7 cm in size
Multiple short segments with normal or 'skipped' area in between
These "skip" lesions are characteristics of AA
Diffuse involvement
May be continuous or with a stretch of normal area in between.

Changes in the aortic lumen
Due to intimal involvement
4 types of changes are present
Irregular lumen due to large raised intimal plaques
Ectasia
Due to destruction of media
Obstructive lesion
Hallmark of the disease
Due to circumferential intimal thickening
Mainly seen in distal thoracic aorta or abdominal aorta in the region of renal arteries.
Almost never seen in ascending aorta
Aneurysms
Rupture of aneurysms is uncommon due to thick and fibrous adventitia

Lesions: Purely stenotic: 85%, purely dilatative: 2% and mixed: 13%. *Dissection of aorta is rarely seen in AA*

* Only form of aortitis that produces stenosis and occlusion of the aorta. Other forms of inflammatory lesions cause dilatation of the aorta

Extent of involvement
May start from aortic valve and distally it does not extend beyond the origin of inferior mesenteric artery in most cases. Rarely in diffuse involvement of abdominal aorta, the lesion may extend up to bifurcation of aorta or even beyond to the common iliac arteries.
*Inferior mesenteric artery is the maximally spared vessel amongst the aortic branches

Pattern of involvement

In Aorta
Ascending Aorta:
May be spared altogether or minimal involvement
Rarely aneurysm formation or Annuloaortic ectasia (involving aortic valve) is seen

*Distinctly different from other inflammatory conditions of aorta where ascending aorta is the primarily involved

Arch of Aorta

Descending thoracic aorta
Frequent in India

May involve ostium of left subclavian artery (LSCA) and extends up to mid thoracic level, usually ends as a stenotic lesion

May start distal to origin of LSCA (ostium is spared) and extends up to level of diaphragm, usually ends as a stenotic lesion

Abdominal aorta

Starts at the level of celiac and ends little proximal to inferior mesenteric artery

Most severe lesions in the region of renal arteries

Renal artery stenosis is common even in non obstructive involvement of abdominal aorta

In aortic branches

Renal and subclavian arteries are most commonly affected

Intercostal arteries affection is even more common but it is not clinically significant

Nature of lesion

Ostial involvement is most common

Arteritis of the branch leading to stenosis or occlusion with or without ostial lesion is less common

Arch vessels

Affects distal part more than the proximal part

Subclavian: 40 %

Right innominate: 7.5 %

Compared to other aortic branches where only a proximal centimeter or two is involved, the disease in arch vessels is more extensive and may spare the ostium.
Lesions may extend up to axillary arteries

Renal arteries

Ostial lesion most common (60 %)
Complete block (38 %)
Bilateral involvement more common (2.5 times) than unilateral involvement

Coronary arteries

Ostial and proximal involvement more common
Rarely distal involvement
Ectasia is rarely seen; mainly stenotic lesions
Only epicardial arteries are involved

Clinical Manifestation

Onset of disease:
    Insidious   76%
    Sudden   24%

Subsequent **course of the disease**
    Plateau crescendo   40%
    Plateau   36%
    Decrescendo   19%
    Decrescendo plateau crescendo 5%

Gender distribution
    More common in females
        More evident in Japanese and Maxican studies
    Indian studies: Males more affected
        Panja et al: M: F = 6.4: 1
        Padmawati et al: M: F = 1.3: 1

Clinical features of active disease

    Fever   20 - 42 %
    Loss of Weight   More than 4.5 kg in 36 % cases (Hall et al)
    Arthragia and Arthritis
        About 50 % cases
        Das et al reported 10.9 % incidence
    Fatigue and Generalized weakness: 34 % (Nakao et al)
    Night sweat and Anorexia: 7 % (Nakao et al)
    Skin rash

Pleuritic chest pain

Lynphadenopathy: Cervical and axillary nodes

Tenderness over the affected vessel

Myocarditis: Reported by Arora et al and Talwar et al (8 out of 11 cases)

Seen in active disease

Pericarditis and tamponade: Rare

Haemoptysis and cough

Exertional breathlessness.

Cerebrovascular accident

Chronic phase:-Obstructive changes are more common

Obstructive changes

Diminished pulse,

Bruit,

Local ischemia,

High BP and difference in BP of both arms.

Clinical Features:
Specific organ involvement

Cardiovascular System
Linkage with HLA Bw52 antigen

Hypertension: Common; seen in 78 % cases

Etiology
Renal artery stenosis
Atypical aortic Coarctation
Reduced aortic capacitance
Abnormal Baroreceptor reactivity

Usually mild to moderate in severity (44 %) than severe (32 %)

May be difficult to diagnose due to occlusive changes in aorta and its branches

Severity
Mild:
Brachial: 140 – 159 / 90 – 94 mm Hg
Popliteal: 160 – 179 / 90 – 94 mm Hg

Moderate:
Brachial: 160 – 199 / 95 – 109 mm Hg
Popliteal: 180 – 229 / 95 – 109 mm Hg

11

Severe:
Brachial: > 200 / 110 mm Hg
Popliteal: > 230 / 110 mm Hg

Congestive heart failure (CHF): Seen in about 28 % cases

Causes
Hypertension
Myocarditis and dilated cardiomyopathy
Valvular regurgitation (AR and MR)
Coronary (ostial lesion) involvement

Myocarditis
Seen in active disease
Common cause of CHF

Dilated cardiomyopathy: 5-20%
Chronic stage

Due to
Systemic hypertension
Valvular regurgitant lesions
Isolated cardiomyopathy

Common cause of DCM in young Indian subsets

Valvular involvement

Aortic regurgitation: Rare; 7 - 24 %
Aortic dilation with separation of aortic commissures
Valve involvement due to extension of aortitis
Annuloaortic ectasia (Annulus dilation with valve involvement)
Usually requires Bentall's procedure

Mitral regurgitation: 3.1 – 11 %
MV prolapse is common
MV deformity is rare
Also due to LV dilatation

Coronary artery involvement
8 – 10 %
Mainly ostial stenotic lesions
Coronary aneurysm is rare

Decrease or absent pulse: 96 %
Bruit: 94 %

Pulmonary artery involvement

Seen in 15 –27 % patients in Indian series
AA is the only form of aortitis to involve pulmonary arteries
Lobar, segmental or sub-segmental pulmonary artery branches are involved
Upper lobe more common than lower lobe
Right lung more common than left (Sharma et al; 72.8 %, Panja et al; 87.5 %)
Typically stenosis or occlusion of branches
Dilatation of main pulmonary artery (MPA) or its branches are **rare**

Multiple sites of involvement is more common

Symptoms and signs

    Chest pain

    Hemoptysis,

    Pleural effusion

    Features of Pulmonary hypertension.

    Mid systolic murmur or vascular bruits may be present

Extensive collateral circulation is seen (PA to bronchial, inferior phrenic, intercostal or coronary artery)

Dieulofoy's lesion: Abnormal submucosal artery in GI tract

    Associated with PA involvement

Central Nervous System: 22.5 -40%

Headache

Syncope

Hemiplegia

Visual disturbances

    Related to hypertension or cerebral ischemia

Eye Changes – Seen up to 52 % of cases

Description of Takayasu (Japanese ophthalmologist 1908): Reported following findings in a 21 yrs old female

    – Peculiar flush in ocular fundi

    – 'Wreath' like AV anastomosis around papilla

    – Blindness due to cataract

The spectrum of eye changes in AA can be classified into:

Hypertensive Retinopathy
>Arteriosclerotic retinopathy
>>Arteriolar narrowing
>>AV nipping
>>Silver wiring

>Neuroretinopathy
>>Hemorrhage
>>Exudates
>>Papilledema

>Hypertensive changes
>>AA Vs Coarctation of Aorta:
>>"corkscrew" arteries in coarctation of Aorta.

Ischemic Retinopathy
>Classified by Uyama and Asayama
>>Stage I: Dilatation of small vessels
>>Stage II: Microaneurysm
>>Stage III: AV anastomosis
>>Stage IV: Ocular complication

Mixed retinopathy

Prognostic Implication of eye involvement:

Eye changes are related to overall disease severity
>Stage I
>>Indicates mild to moderate form of disease
>> Stage II
>>Occurs only if arch vessel lesions are severe and extensive

Patients

Without major complication of TA show retinopathy in 9.4 %,

With 2 or more complication show retinopathy in more than 50 %

Those without carotid artery involvement show retinopathy in 18 %

With severe bilateral carotid artery disease show retinopathy in more than 80 %

Indian characteristics of AA

Association with Tuberculosis (Kinare)

Association with HLA B5/B21 (Kumar, 1990)

Pathology: Increased incidence of aneurysm formation
  (Balakrishnan 18%)

Sex: More male preponderance
  M/F: 1:1.6 (Khallilulah / Balakrishnan)
  Vs Japan/Mexico: 1: 9.7 and SE Asia: 1:2.2

Acute phase or initial systemic illness is very rarely seen in India

Myocarditis and Cardiomyopathy were described as causative
  factor of CHF (first from India)

Classification of Aortoarteritis

Classification: Angiographic

Type I: Localized to aortic arch and its branches (Figure I)

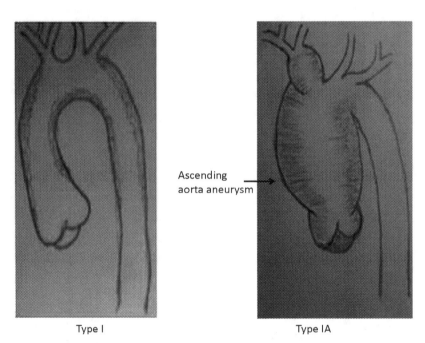

Ascending aorta aneurysm

Type I

Type IA

Figure I type 1

Type II: Thoraco-abdominal aorta and branches without aortic arch involvement (Figure IIA)

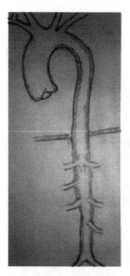

Figure IIA

Type III: Combination of Type I and II (Figure IIB)

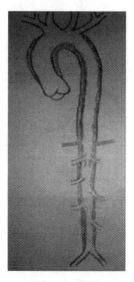

Figure IIB

Commonest in Indian series (also in western; Lupin – 65%)
- Balakrishnan – 52 %
- Kallilulah-   53%

Type IV: Pulmonary artery involvement (Figure III)
- Balakrishnan- 5 %, Kallilulah- 26%, Lupin- 45%

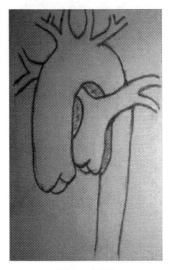

Figure III

Type V: Coronary artery involvement
- Balakrishnan- 6 %, Lupin- 10%

Proposed by
    Ueno (1967):   Types I, II and III
    Lupi-Herrera (1975): IV
    Ottoa: V

Incidence of different types:

Type	North India (Agarwal et al)	East India (Panja et al)	Mexican
I	22%	16%	8%
II	25%	8%	11%
III	**53%**	**76%**	65%
IV	26%	36%	45%
V	10%		

Classification: Clinical

Proposed by Balakrishnan
    Group I: Uncomplicated
    Group II: Mono-complicated
      A: Mild to moderate degree
      B: Severe complication

    Group III: Multicomplicated

    Major complications: Hypertension, Retinopathy, Aortic regurgitation and Aneurysm

Classification: Aortography

Proposed by Nasu

    Type 1: Involvement of the branches of aortic arch only
    Type 2: Involvement of the thoracic aorta and its branches
    Type 3: Involvement of abdominal aorta and its branches
    Type 4: Extensive involvement of whole length of aorta and its branches

Investigations

Acute phase Reactants

    Mild leucocytosis

    Anemia of chronic disease: Normocytic and normochromic

    ESR > 40 mm / hr - after one hour

    Increase in ASO Titre or CRP

    Elevated levels of immunoglobins: IgG, IgA, IgM levels are high
        in 50 % cases

    Circulating immune complex: seen in 50 % cases but no relation
        with disease activity

    Positive RA factor, ANF and elevated levels of fibrinogen
        (Braunwald)

    Positive ANCA

    Urine

        Proteinuria

        Albuminuria

X-ray chest:-

    Described by Ishikawa

        Widening of aortic knob

        Thoracic aortic irregularity

        Decrease pulmonary vascularity (Focal)

        Aortic calcification

Other findings

Cardiomegaly

Rib notching: Not seen in routine cases as ostia of intercostals arteries are affected (compare with Coarctation of aorta)

If thoracic aorta is spared and LSCA block is present; rib notching may be present in first 2-3 ribs

Notching of lower ribs suggest abdominal aorta stenosis or occlusion

X-Ray Abdomen:

Aortic irregularity and calcification

Catheterization and angiography:

DSA is the most important tool

Pan-aortography is required to know the extent and severity of disease

Coronary angiography and pulmonary angiography should also be performed

Special attention to arch vessels

Angulated view may be required to diagnose ostial lesions

Lateral view in abdominal aorta to diagnose involvement of its major branches

Femoral approach may be used in most patients even if the pulse is not palpable (fills up from collaterals); in rare cases of total aortic occlusion, upper limb approach may be required. In extreme cases where arterial approach is not possible, transseptal puncture may be required to do an anterograde angiography.

Findings on angiography:

Luminal irregularities, stenosis and dilatation
"Rat tail appearance": Involvement of the thoracic aorta and
its branches (Nasu Type 2). (Figure IV)

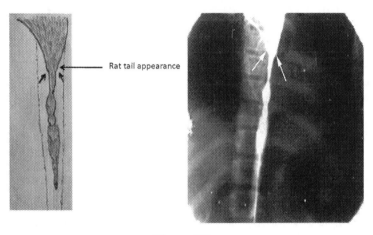

Figure IV

Collateral flow and extent of disease
Endomyocardial biopsy is rarely required these days

Ultrasonography:

High resolution **B mode ultrasonography**
Intimal – medial thickening in carotid arteries

IVUS (Intravascular Ultrasound)
Thickening and altered echogenicity of media
Adventitia and periarterial involvement can be detected as
vessel may appear normal in such cases on angiography

Echocardiography
    Detects valvular pathology and severity
    LV function and dimensions
    Myocarditis
    Helpful in detecting ascending and descending aortic involvement
        TEE is more useful

Spiral CT and CT Angiography:

Useful in evaluating aortic and pulmonary involvement
Coronary evaluation is also possible

MRI scan

Bright signals of edema in and around inflamed vessel
Thickening, obstruction, dilatation and calcification of affected
    vessels.
Mural involvement and thrombi can be detected

Contrast MRI scan

Enhancement of vessel suggests edema, indicative of **acute phase**

Diagnosis of Aortoarteritis

Clinical criteria: Ishikawa

Sign & Symptoms of ≥ 1 month duration

Obligatory criteria: Age ≤ 40 yrs

Major criteria
  Pulselessness or pulse differences in the limbs
  An unobtainable BP
  BP difference in arms > 10 mmHg
  Easy fatigability or pain

Minor criteria:
  Unexplained fever or high ESR
  Neck pain
  Transient amaurosis or blurred vision or syncope
  Dyspnea, palpitation or both

Clinical Diagnosis

Obligatory criteria: Age: ≤ 40 yrs at diagnosis or at onset of "characteristic sign & symptoms" of 1 month duration in patient's history

Diagnosis in presence of obligatory criteria with 2 major criteria or 1 major and ≥ 2 minor criteria or ≥ 4 minor criteria

Ishikawa Criteria: Consists of 1 obligatory, 2 major and 9 minor criteria

Criterion   Definition

Obligatory Criteria

    Age ≤ 40 Yrs   Age ≤ 40 yr at diagnosis or at the onset of 'characteristic signs and symptoms' of 1 month duration in patient history

Two major criteria

1. Left mid subclavian artery lesion

    The most severe stenosis or occlusion present in mid portion from the point 1 cm proximal to the left vertebral artery orifice to that 3 cm distal to the orifice determined by angiography

2. Right mid subclavian artery lesion

    The most severe stenosis or occlusion present in mid portion from the point 1 cm proximal to the right vertebral artery orifice to that 3 cm distal to the orifice determined by angiography

Nine minor criteria

1. High ESR:

    Unexplained persistent high ESR ≥ 20 mm/h (Westergren) at diagnosis or presence of evidence in patient history

2. Carotid artery tenderness:

> Unilateral or bilateral tenderness of common carotid arteries by palpation: neck muscles tenderness is unacceptable

3. Hypertension:

> Persistent blood pressure ≥ 140/90 mm Hg brachial or ≥ 160/90 mm Hg popliteal at age ≤ 40 yr or presence of the history at age ≤ 40 yr

4. Aortic regurgitation

> By auscultation or Doppler echocardiography or angiography

or Annuloaortic ectasia

> By angiography or 2 D echocardiography

5. Pulmonary artery lesion

> Lobar or segmental arterial occlusion or equivalent determined by angiography or perfusion scintigraphy; or presence of stenosis, aneurysm, luminal irregularity, or any combination in pulmonary trunk or in unilateral or bilateral pulmonary arteries determined by angiography

6. Left mid common carotid lesion:

> Presence of the most severe stenosis or occlusion in the mid portion of 5 cm in length from point 2 cm distal to its orifice determined by angiography

7. Distal Brachiocephalic trunk lesion:
>   Presence of the most severe stenosis
>   or occlusion in the distal third
>   determined by angiography

8. Descending thoracic aorta lesion
>   Narrowing, dilation or aneurysm,
>   luminal irregularity, or any
>   combination determined by
>   angiography: tortuosity alone is
>   unacceptable

9. Abdominal aorta lesion.
>   Narrowing, dilation or aneurysm,
>   luminal irregularity, or any
>   combination and absence of lesion
>   in aortoiliac region consisting of 2
>   cm of terminal aorta and bilateral
>   common iliac arteries determined
>   by angiography: tortuosity alone is
>   unacceptable

High probability of TA is suggested if in addition to obligatory criteria.

Two major criteria or **One major** and **two or more minor** criteria or **Four** or more **minor** criteria are present

Criticism
>   Greater applicability in population where arch involvement
>   is more common as major criteria relate to it

American College of Rheumatology (ACR) Criteria for diagnosis of AA: 6 criteria

Criterion	Definition
1. Age at disease onset <40yrs	Development of symptoms or findings related to Takayasu's arteritis at age ≤ 40 yr
2. Claudication of extremities:	Development and worsening of fatigue and discomfort in muscles of one or more extremities while in use, especially the upper extremities
3. Decrease brachial artery pulse	Decreased pulsation of one or both brachial arteries
4. BP difference > 10 mm Hg	Difference of > 10 mm Hg in systolic blood pressure between arms
5. Bruit over subclavian arteries or aorta	Bruit audible on auscultation over one or both subclavian arteries or abdominal aorta
6. Arteriogram abnormality	Arteriographic narrowing or occlusion of the entire aorta, its primary branches or large arteries in the proximal upper or lower extremities, not due to arteriosclerosis, fibromuscular dysplasia or similar causes; changes usually focal or segmental.

Presence of three or more criteria favors TA

Criticism

Less specific

Hypertension (a common symptom) is not included

Ectatic lesions, pulmonary or coronary lesions are not included

Sharma's Criteria

Sharma BK et al, Int J Cardiol 1996; 54 Suppl S 141 - 7

Three Major

1. Right mid subclavian artery lesion
2. Left mid subclavian artery lesion
3. Characteristic signs and symptoms of more than 1 month duration

Ten Minor criteria

High ESR,

Carotidynia,

High Blood Pressure,

Aortic regurgitation,

Annuloaortic ectasia,

Pulmonay artery lesion,

Left mid common carotid lesion,

Distal brachiocephalic lesion,

Descending thoracic aorta lesion,

Abdominal aorta lesion and

Coronary artery lesion.

Two Major or one major and two minor or four minor criteria suggest high probability of TA.

Modifications includes
1. Removal of obligatory criteria
2. Inclusion of characteristic signs and symptoms as major criteria
3. Removal of age in defining HBP
4. Deletion of absence of aorto-illiac lesion
5. Addition of coronary artery lesion

	Sensitivity	Specificity
Sharma	92.5 %	95 %
Ishikawa	60.9 %	95 %

Natural history of Aortoarteritis

Variable

Slowly progressive disease

Presence of one or more of four major complications (hypertension, retinopathy, aneurysm formation and aortic regurgitation) has shown to affect prognosis.

(See study from Balakrishnan et al)

Aortoarteritis: Special subsets

AA in children
Youngest age reported
2 yr: Talwar et al
5 yr: Panja et al

Characteristic features:
Early and uncomplicated lesions are more common

Demarcation between diseased segment and normal segment
(skip lesion) is very distinct

Localized disease is more frequent in children

Localized disease is equally common in thoracic and
abdominal aorta in children whereas in adults is it more
common in abdominal aorta

Main presenting features
Systemic hypertension:
Most common cause of HT in south Asian children
Usually mild to moderate in severity
Obstructive aortoarteritis
Congestive heart failure
More common than adults
Intractable and responds poorly to medical treatment
Severe cachexia with symptoms of immunodeficiency
Risk of sudden death is high

Stenosis more common that aneurysm formation (15 – 20% only)

Renal artery is the most common branch to involve (60-75%) followed by subclavian vessels (41 – 67 %)

Some series have found higher incidence of hypertensive encephalopathy and neurological deficits

Management

Steroids is the main stay of treatment

Immunosuppressants are not commonly used

Balloon angioplasty

Effective

Higher restenosis rate

AA and pregnancy

Basic disease (active or inactive stage) is not modified by gestation

Fertility is not affected by AA

Cardiovascular complications are enhanced

Accelerated and uncontrolled hypertension can lead to

Pre – eclampsia

Congestive heart failure

Renal failure

Antepartum hemorrhage

Intracerebral hemorrhage has been described during labour (each uterine contraction can increase SBP by 20 – 75 mm Hg)

If AA is treated well the outcome of pregnancy is usually favorable

Fetal outcome

Higher incidence of IUGR: Due to

Poor control of blood pressure

CHF

Delay in seeking medical advice

Decreased placental flow (Abdominal aorta involvement)

Management

Steroids are safe in pregnancy

Labor:

Vaginal delivery is preferred

Cut short the second stage of labor

Aortoarteritis: Management

Before deciding the management strategies, it is essential to rule out active phase of disease. The active phase has bearing upon the treatment decision. National Institute Of Health has defined following criteria for diagnosis of active disease.

New onset or worsening of at least 2 of the following 4 features:
1. Sign and symptoms of vascular ischemia or inflammation (e.g., claudication, decreased or absent extremity pulses or blood pressure or carotidynia)
2. Elevated erythrocyte sedimentation rate (ESR)
3. Angiographic abnormalities
4. Systemic symptoms not attributable to another disease.

Management of aortoarteritis depends on clinical presentation and activity of the disease.

Medical therapy

Recommended to
Patients with active and / or lesions not in need of surgical or non surgical intervention
Patients in whom surgical or non surgical intervention are not feasible or at a very high risk because of comorbid conditions.
Patients who refuse surgical or non surgical intervention

Medical therapy is based on clinical symptomatology and immunological basis of disease. In absence of exact etiology, specific treatment is not available.

Symptomatic treatment:
   Antihypertensive medications:
      Vasodilators are preferred
   Treatment for congestive heart failure
      Regular antifailure treatment as per need of patient
   Treatment of ischemia symptoms
   Antiplatelets and anticoagulants are used: Efficacy is not well established

Treatment for Control of active disease:

Corticosteroids
   Prednisolone: 1 mg / kg / day
      Tapered to an alternative day regimen after 3 months of daily therapy. Dose should be tapered to a minimum level to keep ESR within normal limits
   Monitoring of treatment efficacy:
      Weekly ESR
      Improvement in sign and symptoms of vascular ischemia or inflammation

Cytotoxic therapy:
   Drugs used
      Cyclophosphamide: 2 mg / kg / day
      Azathioprine: 100 mg / day
      Methotrexate (low dose / week) in combination with steroids

Indications:

Progression of disease on steroid therapy

Steroids cannot be tapered to alternate day regimen in 3 months

Aortoarteritis associated with myocarditis (diagnosed by endomyocardial biopsy)

Role of antitubecular treatment

Proposed by Sen et al, based on findings in 52 patients.

At present there is **no** role of empirical antitubercular treatment.

Surgical or Non surgical Treatment:

Indications:

1. Hypertension from stenotic coarctation of aorta or renovascular disease
2. End-organ ischemia or peripheral limb ischemia
3. Aneurysm formation

Non surgical management

Percutaneous Transluminal Balloon Angioplasty (PTBA) with or without stenting

Advantages over conventional surgical techniques:

Effective

Less invasive

Safe

Stenting is associated with excellent angiographic and clinical results. Stenting should be avoided in active disease.

PTBA of Aortic involvement

Highly effective for discrete lesions

Less effective for long segment, eccentric or calcific lesions

Stents:

Self expanding stents: Available in long length and large diameters

Wall stent

Memotherm stent

Balloon expandable stents

Covered stent graft

Useful for aneurysms

Caution:

Often require high inflation pressure for dilation as lesions of aortoarteritis are rigid. Special care should be taken to avoid rupture and aneurysm formation.

PTBA for Renal lesions:

Lesions characteristics:

Ostial or proximal segment involvement

Fibrotic and calcific lesions

More effective for discrete lesions

As in other lesions of aortoarteritis, higher inflation pressure (4-17 bars versus 2-6 bars in atherosclerotic lesions) are required to dilate the lesion

Improvement in hypertension is seen in 80 – 90 % cases

Restenosis:
    16 – 22 % in adults
    20 – 26 % in children

Stents have improved the outcome of PTBA (Tietmeyer et al, Arora et al)
Success rate: 95 – 99 %
Long term patency rate: 84 % at 5 yr follow up
Restenosis: 10 – 12 %

PTBA of Arch Vessels:

Subclavian artery lesions:
    Primary success rate: 73 – 100 %
        Low success rate in total occlusion
        Restenosis more common with
            Long segment lesions
            Diffuse vascular narrowing
            Partial or suboptimal dilation
            Active disease state
    Complication rate: 0-10 %
Carotid and vertebral artery lesions:
    Safer than atherosclerotic lesions
    Less chance of embolic episodes because of inflammatory and non ulcerative lesions of aortoarteritis

PTBA of Mesenteric or Iliac arteries
    Inferior mesenteric artery is usually spared in aortoarteritis
    Celiac and superior mesenteric lesions are amenable to PTBA/stenting treatment
    Highly successful for iliac artery lesions also

Coronary artery lesions:
Isolated reports

Surgical treatment   Options:

Bypass of the obstructed arteries

Resection of the narrowed segment and replacement with an interposition graft

Patch aortoplasty for short segment lesion

Endarterectomy

Excision of saccular aneurysm

Rarely aortic valve replacement with or without aortic root replacement

Challenges:
High mortality rate
High complication rates
Graft occlusions
Anastomotic site aneurysms

Techniques for renal artery lesions
Aorto-renal bypass grafts (Saphenous vein or PTFE)
Direct aortic reimplantation
Thromboendarterectomy

Abdominal visceral arteries:
Endarterectomy for osteal lesions
Prosthetic bypass for distal lesions

Aortoarteritis: Important Indian Studies

Natural History of Aortoarteritis
Subramanyam, Balakrishnan et al
Circ 1989; 80: 429-37

n= 88 (M 34)
Age (at onset of symptoms): 24.0±8.8 yrs
Follow–up: 83.6±74.4 months (from onset)
Total deaths: 10 (11.4%): 0.16 death per patient year
Four groups
Group I: Uncomplicated
Group II: Mono-complicated
    A: Mild to moderate degree
    B: Severe complication
Group III: Multi-complicated

Major complications: Hypertension, Retinopathy, Aortic
regurgitation and Aneurysm

Severity of HT as defined in clinical features
AR:
    Severe if grade III – IV on angiography
Retinopathy
    Mild to moderate: Stage I – II
    Severe: Stage III - IV
Aneurysm was considered severe in the diameter was
more than 2 times normal diameter

Survival:

Group	Event-free (5yrs)	10 yrs
I/IIA	97%	97%
IIB/III	60%	39%

Cumulative survival
5 yrs: 91±3.3 %
10 yrs: 84±5.6%

Predictors of death or major event
Severe hypertension
Evidence of cardiac involvement
Severe functional disability

Congestive cardiomyopathy in non specific aortoarteritis
Arora, Sethi KK et al
J Assoc Physicians India 1985; 33: 333-335
n=120
Occurrence of primary myocardial involvement in NSAA was emphasized
Cases with cardiomyopathy: 7
Normal coronaries
Normal pulmonary arteries

Pulmonary artery involvement in aortoarteritis
Tyagi S, Khallilulah M et al
Ind Heart J 1987; 39: 415 – 19

Pulmonary artery involvement in AA (By pulmonary angiography)
n=38
PA involvement: 10 (26%)
Pulmonary arterial hypertension (23.7%)
Occlusion was commonest in right upper lobe artery

Cardiac involvement in non specific aortoarteritis
Talwar KK, Tandon R et al
Am Heart J 1991; 122 (6): 1666-70

n=44

Emphasized that myocardial involvement including myocarditis is common in NSAA

Lesions	n
Hypertension	35
CHF	24 (high as compared to other series)
MR	6
AR	2
Raised RA pressure	9 ($\geq$ 7 mmHg)
Raised PA pressure (mean)	29 ($\geq$ 20 mm Hg)
Raised LV filling pressure	27
Decreased LVEF (<45%)	27
Left main stenosis	1

Balloon angioplasty of the Aorta in Takayasu's arteritis: Initial and long term results
Tyagi S, Arora R et al
Am Heart J 1992; 124: 876-882

n=36

Age: 8-36 yrs

Success: 34 (95%)

Success indicators: Short segment (<4cm)

No significant complications (No aneurysm ? Due to panarteritis)

Follow-up: 3-24 months

Restenosis: 1

Requires very high balloon inflation pressure as compared to atherosclerotic disease; as the aorta is very rigid

Balloon angioplasty for renovascular hypertension in Takayasu's arteritis
Tyagi S, Khalilullah M et al
Am Heart J 1993; 125: 1386 – 1393

n=54 (75 lesions)
Success: 89.3%
HT decreases within 48 hrs. in successful cases. BP either was normal or improved in 93% of successful cases.
Follow-up: 26.4±10.3 (3-70 months)
Restenosis: 13.5% at the same site
Balloon size is equal to estimated original diameter of artery at the stenosed area.

Aortoarteritis and tuberculosis
The association suggested by Kinare et al appears to be coincidental

The differentiating points from Tuberculous aortitis

	Takayasu's Arteritis	Tuberculous Aortitis
Extent	Localized or diffuse	Localized
Dominant lesion	Stenosis	Dilatation
Aneurysms	Multiple (Fusiform/ saccular/ dissecting)	Single (Saccular)
Histopathology	Proliferative and Non caseating granuloma	Caseating granuloma

Focus of infection	Not always in paraaortic region	Commonly in paraaortic region
Mycobacterium	Not cultured	Cultured

Ruptured Sinus Of Valsalva

Ruptured Sinus of Valsalva (RSOV)

John Thurnam first described sinus of Valsalva aneurysm (SVA) in 1840. A detailed description was written by Hope in 1939.

Incidence:

> Uncommon in western countries
>> Common in Asian countries
>
> 1.1 - 0.35 % of congenital heart disease (CHD)

Anatomy of Sinus of Valsalva (SOV)

> The 3 sinuses of Valsalva are located in the most proximal portion of the aorta, just above the cusps of the aortic valve. The sinuses correspond to the individual cusps of the aortic valve. These structures contained within the pericardium are easily revealed using aortography and echocardiography as distinct, but subtle, out-pouching of the aortic wall just above the valve cusps. The sinuses end in the area of the sinotubular junction, and the tubular portion of the aorta begins here.

Pathology of Aneurysm of Sinus of Valsalva (ASOV)

Aneurysm of SOV can be localized or diffuse. Diffuse involvement may involve multiple sinuses or entire aorta. Localized involvement is seen with congenital causes. Diffuse involvement may be seen with both congenital and acquired causes.

Localized or diverticular aneurysms of SOV

Mode of development of ASOV: The various 'theories'

Proposed by Abbott: Abnormal development of the bulbus cordis
The basic cause is incomplete fusion of conus ridges:
The incomplete fusion leads to fragile tissue at the local site. Although the defect is inherited, but frank aneurysmal dilatation is rarely seen at birth. Aneurysms typically develop as a discrete flaw in the aortic media within one of the sinuses of Valsalva. The site is prone to dilation due to high blood pressure (diverticular aneurysm) or high blood pressure and infective endocarditis (irregular diverticular aneurysm). Lack of supporting tissue (e.g., ventricular septal defect) may contribute to instability and progressive

distortion of the aortic sinus, often with associated aortic insufficiency. Rupture of ASOV results due to progressive dilatation caused by high blood pressure acting on a weak point in the aortic wall. In rare cases the local point may rupture into muscular septum leading to hematoma and formation of pseudoaneurysm.

> *As only right coronary cusp. (RCC) and non-coronary cusp. (NCC) are related to bulbar septum; explains the fact that most ASOVs are related to these cusps only.*

Proposed by Venning:

ASOV is due to local defect of elastic tissue at the base of aorta.

Proposed by Edwards:

Separation of aortic media and annulus fibrosis of aortic valve.

The bulbar septum theory explains the most of the cases of ASOV and also the ventricular septal defect (VSD) associated with ASOVs. However, ASOV related to LCC (left coronary cusp) although rare cannot be explained by this theory. But cases where ASOVs are related to LCC, the evidence that points to their congenital origin is not convincing.

Diffuse ASOV

Congenital causes
  Marfan syndrome,
  Ehlers-Danlos syndrome,
  Turner syndrome,
  Williams syndrome,
  Bicuspid aortic valve,
  Coarctation of Aorta, and
  Osteogenesis imperfecta

Mode of development
  Medionecrosis
    Seen in Marfan syndrome and in similar syndromes
    Weakness in medial layer leads to diffuse fragile tissue.
      With high blood pressure there is diffuse aneurysmal dilatation of aorta.
    * Approximately 10% of patients with Marfan syndrome have some form of ASOV
  Underdevelopment of elastic tissue: It also leads to diffuse fragile tissue and diffuse aneurysm formation as in medionecrosis.

  In few cases the exact defect is not known and the common precipitating factor is high blood pressure (seen in cases of coarctation of aorta)

Acquired causes:

  Infections of ascending aorta
    Tuberculosis, syphilis or infective endocarditis

Due to infection the aortic wall becomes weak. High blood pressure in such cases leads to development of aneurysm with irregular margins and shape.

Other causes include
Atherosclerosis
Blunt or penetrating chest injuries

Jones and Langley list the following criteria for differentiating the 2 types.
JONES, A. M., AND LANGLEY, F. A.: Aortic sinus aneurysm. BHJ. 11: 325, 1949

In the congenital type, the aneurysm
   (1) Is confined to the right coronary sinus and adjacent two thirds of the noncoronary sinus;
   (2) Is usually small;
   (3) Commonly ruptures into the right ventricle or right atrium;
   (4) Remains intracardiac;
   (5) Is usually associated with other developmental defects.

In the acquired type, the aneurysm
   (1) May arise from any sinus;
   (2) Tends to extend upward;
   (3) Is often extacardiac;
   (4) Cardio-aortic fistulae are rare;
   (5) Congenital cardiac defects are rare;
   (6) It is always associated with acquired heart disease, usually syphilis or bacterial endocarditis

Associated structural defects in congenital ASOVs

Supracristal or perimembranous ventricular septal defect (30-60%),
Bicuspid aortic valve (15-20%) and
Aortic regurgitation (44-50%).
Less commonly observed anomalies
Pulmonary stenosis,
Coarctation, and
Atrial septal defects

Classification of ASOV

<u>Japanese Classification</u>

1. Sinus of Valsalva from which aneurysm arises (Figure I)
   RCC
   NCC

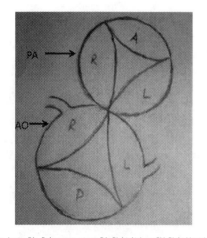 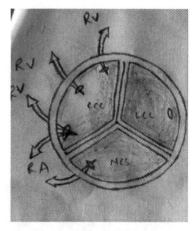

AO: Aorta, PA: Pulmonary artery; RA: Right Atrium; RV: Right Ventricle;
RCC: Right Coronary cusp; LCC: Left Coronary cusp; NCC: Non Coronary cusp;
R: Right cusp; L: Left cusp; A: Anterior cusp; P: Posterior cusp

Figure I

2. Encroached part of SOV: Point of localized involvement
   (Figure I & II)
   RCC
Left:	Type I
Central:	Type II
Posterior:	Type III

NCC

Right: Type IV

3. Direction of protrusion and cardiac chambers into which the aneurysm protrudes (Figure II)

Type I: Into the conus of right ventricle (RV), just beneath the commissure of left and right cusps of pulmonary valve

Type II: Into the body of RV, penetrating crista supraventricularis

Type III:

'v': Into the RV (hence 'v'), just beneath the septal leaflet of tricuspid valve (TV) penetrating the membranous septum

'a': Into the atrium (hence 'a'), near the commissure of septal tricuspid leaflet (STL) and anterior tricuspid leaflet (ATL) of TV.

Type IV: Into the right atrium (RA), near the (STL) of TV

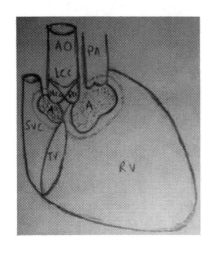 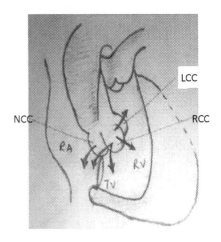

A: Aneurysm; AO: Aorta, PA: Pulmonary artery; RA: Right Atrium; RV: Right Ventricle;
RCC: Right Coronary cusp; LCC: Left Coronary cusp; NCC: Non Coronary cusp;
SVC: Superior Vena Cava; TV: Tricuspid valve

Figure II

4. With or without VSD

Site of VSD
Type I: Just beneath the pulmonary valve (PV) (subpulmonary VSD). Occasional case reports of association of membranous VSD in type I is not explained on embryonic development, association is likely to be coincidental.

Type II: VSD at crista supraventricularis

Type III or IV: Membranous VSD

Sakakibara and Konno Classification
Cardiac Surg Ann 2006;9:165-176

Type I- Right SV & existing tract of RV below pulmonary valve
Type II- Right SV into the supraventricularis crest
Type IIIa- Right SV & RA
Type IIIv- Posterior zone of right SV & RV
Type IIIa+v- Right SV & both RA and RV
Type IV- Noncoronary SV & RA

Chinese classification (Shanghai chest hospital classification)

Simple classification based on anatomical findings. Subgroups based on whether ASOV is ruptured or unruptured.

Based on a study of 105 cases
1. Aneurysm of Valsalva (38 cases)
   Ruptured

      Unruptured

2. ASOV with VSD (48 cases)

      Ruptured

      Unruptured

3. ASOV with aortic regurgitation (AR) (3 cases)

      Ruptured

      Unruptured

4. ASOV with VSD and AR (16 cases)

      Ruptured

      Unruptured

Incidence of various types of ASOV or RSOVs

ASOV arising from RCC: Most common and seen in 75 – 85 %
                      cases
ASOV from NCC: Seen in 5 – 15 % cases.
ASOV from LCC: Extremely rare

Site of rupture

ASOV from RCC
    RV is the commonest site, seen in 85 – 95 % cases of rupture
    Rupture into RA is seen in 5 – 15 % cases

ASOV from NCC
    RV rupture is very uncommon (seen in only 2 -5 % cases); in
        rest of cases it ruptures into RA

Uncommon sites of rupture of ASOV: Seen in nearly 1 % cases.
    Pericardium
    Left atrium (LA)
    Left ventricle (LV)
    Interventricular septum (IVS)
    Pulmonary trunk

Site of rupture as seen in different population

Population	Site of rupture (%)	
	RV	RA
Asian	84	13
Non Asian	57	37
Overall	72	23

Incidence of RSOV (in different series)

Type	Japanese Series (%) (Sakakibara et al) (n=52)	Chinese Series (%) (Guo and Gu et al) (n=105)
I	40 - 45	64.5
With VSD	80	66.7
II	6	22.3
IIIv	8	1.1
IIIa	20 – 25	6.4
IV	20 – 25	3.2

In both series, more than 95 % of ASOV involved either right or non coronary cusp.

VSD was rare except in Type I ASOV.

Clinical presentation of sinus of Valsalva aneurysm

1. Patients with unruptured aneurysms

   Usually asymptomatic.

   Unruptured ASOV: Unusual clinical presentation
   Right ventricle outflow tract (RVOT) obstruction
   Tricuspid regurgitation
   Aortic regurgitation
   Coronary occlusion and compression: Angina
   Unexplained arrhythmias
   Complete heart block (CHB): Compression of conduction
   system

2. Sudden massive rupture may occur after strenuous exertion and may be signaled by acute chest or epigastric pain with dyspnea. Symptoms may be confused with those of acute myocardial infarction.
   Most dramatic and prominent clinical presentation

3. Patients with a smaller insidious rupture may be asymptomatic, but small ruptures also may be associated with progressive symptoms of exertional dyspnea and/or chest discomfort from advancing heart failure.

Stages of progression of ASOV: Unruptured ASOV

Depends on the extent of protrusion and left to right shunt across VSD

Stage I: The ASOV does not bulge into RV but nearly covers VSD. Hence although left to right shunt across VSD is present, the shunt volume is not large enough to produce symptoms. Symptoms at this stage is chiefly due to AR, if at all present.

Stage II: The bulge further increases and takes the shape of a hemisphere. The diameter of the bulge is less than ½ of the aortic diameter. Due to further protrusion, the bulge is now seen into RV and it almost covers the whole VSD. Thus the shunt across VSD is not significant but moderate AR is usually present. Till this stage, rupture of ASOV does not occur unless there is associated inflammation

Stage III: The bulge further increases and is now almost spherical in shape. The tip now is larger than the base (hence spherical in shape) and it now completely occludes the VSD throughout systole and diastole. There is no shunt across VSD. The diameter of ASOV is more than ½ of aortic diameter. The bulge in RV can produce murmur due to anatomical RVOT obstruction and compression effects on surrounding structures. Significant AR is associated at this stage.

Clinical presentation:
Ruptured sinus of Valsalva (RSOV)

Depends upon direction and amount of blood flowing through the abnormal intracardiac communication resulting from rupture. Rupture of the aneurysm may occur spontaneously or be precipitated by trauma, exertion or cardiac catheterization. Although site of rupture may vary, the most common site is right sided cardiac chambers. Rupture of the dilated sinus may lead to intracardiac shunting when a communication is established with the right atrium (Gerbode defect [10%]) or directly into the right ventricle (60-90%). Ruptured ASOVs present with specific signs of left to right shunting and they are indistinguishable from coronary arteriovenous fistulas. The signs are machine type continuous murmurs, bounding pulse, palpable thrill along right or left sternal border. It results into acute left and right ventricular overload and commonly progresses to refractory congestive heart failure.

Dyspnea is the most common presenting symptom.

Age

Aneurysm of Sinus of Valsalva (ASOV) usually produces no symptoms until they rupture

Types of RSOV	Age at rupture (mean age) in yrs
I	13 – 41 (29)
II	30

III a and v	11 – 56 (33)
IV	22 – 67 (34)

Usual age of ASOV rupture is 20 – 35 yrs (mean 32). Although, asymptomatic, types associated with VSD can be detected early due to pan systolic murmur (PSM) of VSD.

Gender difference:
Male preponderance, probably related to difference in load demand of heart between the two genders.

Symptoms

Ruptured SVAs progress in three stages described by **Blackshear** Symptoms usually start at the time of rupture and gradually become chronic if not intervened.

Stage I:
Symptoms at the time of rupture: Sudden onset of angina like pain or right upper abdominal pain associated with nausea and vomiting. This usually lasts for an hour.

Stage II
Alleviation of severe symptoms of rupture with subsequent onset of exertional dyspnea and chest discomfort which persists for next 24 hours.

Stage III
Symptoms of congestive heart failure set in patients who survive sudden rupture of ASOV.

Patients with Type I (with or without VSD) behave differently than other types. In type I cases, ASOV is usually associated with VSD. Left to right shunt exists across VSD. In cases where the ASOV has occluded VSD and obliterates the shunt, usually ASOV protrudes into RVOT and simulates pulmonary stenosis. In either of these 2 situations the circulatory forces are altered and the cardiopulmonary forces as a whole are changed to adapt to these abnormal forces (VSD or pulmonary stenosis (PS) like pathology). Hence the rupture of ASOV does not produce severe shock. The typical symptoms of rupture (Phase I) are absent in such cases. In contrast, other types of ASOV (II, III or IV) have severe symptoms at the onset of rupture. In these types there is no adaptation of circulatory system and the effect of rupture is great on cardiopulmonary function leading to NYHA class IV symptoms at the time of rupture.

Signs

The signs are different in different types of ASOV / RSOV and site of murmur in RSOV is characteristic for each type.

Type I:
Without VSD:
Relatively rare
Before rupture:
Systolic murmur at pulmonary area similar to pulmonary stenosis

After rupture:
Loud to and fro murmur with both systolic and diastolic components. Murmur shows different peaks of intensity and intensity of diastolic component is

greater than systolic component. The murmur is best heard over pulmonary valve orifice. Thrill is almost always present, corresponds to murmur and is strongly felt during diastole.

With VSD:

More common

Before rupture:

Murmurs due to VSD and AR (Pansystolic and early diastolic murmurs)

Pansystolic murmur (due to VSD) is best heard at pulmonary area and the early diastolic murmur of AR is best heard at 3rd intercostals space on left intercostal space (LICS).

After rupture:

Similar to as seen in Type I without VSD.

Other types:

Differ from type I as the VSD is not commonly associated with these types. Hence the clinical signs before rupture of ASOV are absent. Marked symptoms and signs are evident at or after rupture.

Type II:

Before rupture

There is no murmur if VSD is not present (VSD is rare all types except type I)

After rupture:

Similar to type I but the site of maximum intensity of murmur is slightly more rightwards as compared to type I.

Type III: Signs depend whether rupture is in the RV (IIIv) or in atrium (IIIa)

III v:

After rupture:

Continuous murmur best heard at the left or right sternal border in 4th intercostal space. The systolic component is more intense than the diastolic component.

III a:

After rupture:

Loud continuous murmur, best heard at lower end of sternum to upper abdomen. Systolic component is very loud and in most cases only systolic thrill is present.

Type IV:

After rupture:

Similar to type III a, but the intensity of murmur is much weaker and thrill is absent in majority.

The systolic component in RSOV murmur is not as loud as diastolic murmur in most cases except in types where rupture occurs in atrium. The intensity of murmur depends on the pressure difference and shunting of blood across RSOV. Due to venturi effect, the pressure in aortic sinuses reaches its peak during diastole and decrease drastically during systole.

Jugular venous pulse (JVP) in RSOV

RSOV to RA

    Mean   Very high (+++)

    A wave   Very high (upper level may not be seen properly)

    V wave   Very high

    X descent   Shallow

    Y descent   Rapid and deep descend

RSOV to RV

    Mean   High (+)

    A wave   High (++)

    V wave   High (can be distinguished clearly from A wave)

    X descent   Rapid and deep descend

    Y descent   Rapid and deep descend

RSOV: Investigations

CXR findings:
Abnormal in more than 80 % cases. Cardiomegaly is the most common finding seen in 90 – 95 % cases. The typical findings are bilateral dilatation of cardiac chambers and intensification of pulmonary markings is striking. Right atrial enlargement (RAE) is seen in 80 % and left atrial enlargement (LAE) seen in 40 % cases. Aortic knob is normal in almost all cases.

ECG findings:
Type I (with or without VSD)
Sinus rhythm
Biventricular hypertrophy with left ventricle (LV) preponderance
Left ventricular hypertrophy (LVH)

Type III and IV:
LVH with diastolic overload of RV (Incomplete RBBB)
Distinctive findings:
Atrioventricular (AV) conduction disturbances
AV block
Increased PR interval
AV nodal rhythm
RBBB
Wenckebach rhythm

Echocardiography

Transthoracic echocardiography (TTE)

Features:

Generalized single sinus enlargement

"Wind-sock" extension of sinus from body and/or apex or otherwise normal aortic sinus when ruptured

Detection of associated defects including ventricular septal defect, bicuspid aortic valve, and aortic insufficiency

Useful views

PLAX

The anterior sinus is right coronary sinus (most commonly affected in ASOV). Aneurysmal dilatation with rupture and resultant continuous color flow is well seen. The posterior sinus in this view is non coronary sinus.

Color flow and Doppler demonstrates a continuous high velocity unidirectional flow through the lesion and is technique of choice to identify RSOV. It confirms the diagnosis if it demonstrates the unidirectional continuous flow from aorta to right heart chamber

Aortic regurgitation can be identified clearly in this view as the jet is directed towards the LV

Perimembranous VSD can be difficult to diagnose as the color jet of RSOV interferes with VSD jet. Turbulent jet of RSOV masks the jet of VSD. Large VSD can be seen as definite defect in IVS.

PSAX

Very useful view

Usually distinguishes the sinus of involvement as the 3 sinuses are clearly delineated in PSAX view

The site of rupture (in cardiac chambers) is better visualized in this view. Right coronary sinus aneurysm and the resultant rupture into RV (RVOT (beneath pulmonary valve), into RV inflow (just above the tricuspid valve) and into body (in between the above 2 sites; similar to supracristal VSD) can be easily identified. The Doppler finding confirms continuous color flow with high gradient flow.

The width of rupture is measured in this view

Rules out PDA

Apical views

Both 4 and 2 chamber view can show sinus of involvement and rupture site of aneurysm can be seen

<u>Suprasternal views</u>

Pandiastolic flow reversal seen in descending aorta due to RSOV

Concomitant severity of aortic regurgitation cannot be determined by flow reversal.

3 D TTE

Three-dimensional TEE is useful to determine the precise shape, size, and location of the defect and help guide percutaneous closure device placement

Contrast echocardiography

A negative contrast effect with agitated saline bubble contrast in the right heart indicates abnormal flow from the aorta to the respective right heart chamber

TEE (Transesophageal Echocardiography)

Useful in confirming the diagnosis

Also an indispensible tool in device closure of RSOV as well as intraoperative surgical closure.

Demonstrates proper device placement, assessment of aortic valve and presence of any residual shunt during device closure of RSOV

Cardiac catheterization and aortography

Useful views

Right anterior oblique (RAO) 30

Postero-anterior (PA)

Left anterior oblique (LAO) 70

Diameter of RSOV can be measured accurately on aortography

Associated VSD is difficult to rule out on aortography

Aortic regurgitation is easier to diagnose on aortography

CT Angio and MRI

Confirms the diagnosis

Precise morphology of RSOV and size of opening are accurately demonstrated

Hemodynamics

Type I

    Pressure tracing similar to pulmonary stenosis
    Right atrial pressure (RAP); increased mean pressure with high
       'a' wave
    Step up of oxygen saturation in RV

Type II and III v

    Pressure tracing not similar to pulmonary stenosis
    High a wave in RAP
    Step up of oxygen saturation in RV

Type III a and IV:
    Very high RAP with high v wave
    Step up of oxygen saturation in RA

Differential Diagnosis

Patent ductus arteriosus (PDA) and Aortopulmonary (AP) window

VSD with AR

Aortic stenosis (AS) with AR

Anomalous origin of left coronary artery from pulmonary artery (ALCAPA)

Pulmonary and systemic arteriovenous (AV) fistula

Rupture of aortic aneurysm into pulmonary artery

Management

Non ruptured ASOV

The optimal management of an asymptomatic, nonruptured aneurysm is less clear because of the absence of a precise natural history. Improvements in surgical technique in the past 15 years have resulted in low complication rates with no early mortality (0%) and low morbidity (4%).

Ruptured ASOV

Medical therapy:
For Congestive Heart Failure (CHF)
For Infective Endocarditis wherever indicated

Surgical therapy

The surgical mortality rate is estimated to be 5% or less

Surgical approaches to RSOV

3 different approaches depending on the repair performed through

1. The chamber into which ASOV has ruptured
2. Aortic root
3. Combined approach: 'Aortocameral' approach

Associated defect:

Severe AR: Aortic valve replacement (AVR) should be done for severe AR or in patients with fibrotic changes in aortic valve.

VSD: Patch closure for large VSD
Direct suture of small VSD

Surgical Care: Prompt surgical therapy is recommended when a ruptured sinus of Valsalva aneurysm is diagnosed. A combined approach from the affected chamber and from inside the aorta is most helpful to allow inspection of the aortic valve and to avoid injury to the coronary vessels. The procedure is described as follows:

The fistula tract from the ruptured aneurysm is closed, and an associated ventricular septal defect is repaired.

The aorta is reunited with the valve annulus either by direct anastomosis or by the interposition of a graft, if required.

Intra operative transesophageal echocardiography (TEE) should establish competency of AV and if required repair should be done to maintain competency of the valve.

Surgery should be performed early (especially in children) so that AV replacement can be avoided.

No consensus exists as to when to perform surgery on a fortuitously discovered unruptured sinus of Valsalva aneurysm.

Serially monitor these patients using echocardiography or MRI to document the size of the aneurysm.

Undertake elective repair of a known sinus of Valsalva aneurysm at the same time as surgical repair of any other intracardiac shunt or defect.

Non Surgical Therapy

Percutaneous, transcatheter closure of a ruptured sinus of Valsalva aneurysm was first described in 1994. It was performed by Cullen et al using a Rashkind umbrella. More recently, a number of occluder devices have been used, especially the Amplatzer device.

Surgical closure of RSOV in cardiopulmonary bypass was the only possible treatment with relatively low perioperative risk (mortality <2%) in the past. Progress in interventional cardiology during recent years and especially introduction of Amplatzer devices to clinical use enable closure of many undesirable vascular connections. For transcatheter closure of RSOV, initially Rashkind umbrella and coils were used. However, coils can be implanted only in cases of minor connections. The effectiveness and safety of ASO (Amplatzer Septal Occluder) and ADO (Amplatzer Duct Occluder) in transcatheter closure of RSOV and other undesirable vascular connections is now confirmed. In case of RSOV when ADO has unstable position, application of ASO can be a better solution due to its bigger retention discs. Using transcatheter closure can avoid possible complications of medial sternotomy and cardiopulmonary bypass. Reduced pain for the patient, absence of surgical scar, shorter hospitalization and convalescence time are also important advantages. Transcatheter treatment may be especially useful in the case of recanalization after previous surgical treatment, when the risk of reoperation is substantially higher. Theoretically there exists the risk of repeated rupture of the sinus of Valsalva, because of the presence of abnormal tissue. On the other hand, epithelialization of the device can make surrounding tissue stronger. These questions remain unanswered; therefore, longer follow-up after such procedures is needed.

The procedure:

Usual access: Right femoral artery and femoral vein.

1. The procedure is usually carried out under general anesthesia with both fluoroscopy and transoesophageal guidance
   Preferred views for fluoroscopy
   Right anterior oblique (30 degree),
   Postero-anterior or
   Left anterior oblique (70 degree)
2. Assess the diameter of the RSOV
3. Cross the RSOV with help of right Judkins coronary catheter and Terumo wire from the aorta and park the wire in the right atrium or pulmonary artery.
4. Exchange the Terumo wire with 0.035 inch/260 cm long Amplatz extrastiff guide wire
5. Snare and take out the Amplatz extrastiff guide wire through femoral vein to create arteriovenous loop.
6. Introduce a 7 or 8 F transseptal AGA sheath (45 or 180 deg) from femoral vein through the ruptured sinus to the ascending aorta.
7. Either Amplatzer Duct Occluder (ADO) or Amplatzer Atrial Septal Occluder (ASO) (both AGA Medical Corp., Plymouth, MN, USA) is selected to close the RSOV. Size is selected, equal or up to 5 mm larger than RSOV orifice diameter. Confirm the placement of device and residual shunt if any under fluoroscopy and TEE guidance

8. Stability of the opened device is confirmed during "Minnesota wiggle" (gentle pulling and pushing of the delivery system). Once the position of the device is considered acceptable, ECG is analyzed and Amplatzer device is released.

9. The TEE and aortography are repeated

Prognosis

The prognosis is poor with progressive aneurysmal dilatation or rupture unless early surgical repair is performed.

Actuarial survival rate for patients with congenital SVA is 95% at 20 years, since most SVAs do not rupture prior to age 20 years.

Unruptured SVA has been observed in serial monitoring up to several years after initial diagnosis, but most unruptured SVAs have been found to progress and rupture.

Untreated SVAs may rupture, and patients with ruptured SVAs die of heart failure (with left-to-right shunting) or endocarditis within 1 year after onset of symptoms of ruptured SVA.

Exceptional survival up to 17 yrs has been reported in literature.

Post surgery, the actuarial 10-year survival rate was 63%.

(Moustafa S, Mookadam F, Cooper L et al. Sinus of Valsalva aneurysms--47 years of a single center experience and systematic overview of published reports. *Am J Cardiol.* Apr 2007. 99:1159-64)

Indian series

Diagnostic feature of ASOV

Krishnaswami, S. John et al (JAPI 1977)

N = 20

Age: 6 – 41 yrs (mean 20 yrs)

Men: 14

Symptoms:

    Sudden onset: 12 / 20 cases

    Chest pain: 8 out of 12 cases

    Duration of symptoms: 2 weeks to 12 yrs

Signs:

Raised JVP:	12 / 20
Signs of CHF:	9/20
Collapsing pulse:	18 / 20
Loud P2:	16 / 20

Murmurs:

    Systolodiastolic murmur at left sternal border: 6

Continuous murmur:	11 /20
Apical MDM:	15 / 20
EDM:	8
Thrill:	16 / 20

ECG:

1st degree heart block:	1
Complete heart block:	1
RVH only:	5
LVH only:	13
Atrial enlargement:	0

Cardiac catheterization:

Origin from RCC:	14 (70 %)
Origin from NCC:	3 (15 %)
Not clear:	3
Rupture into RV:	13 (65 %)
Rupture into RA:	4 (20 %)
Unruptured:	3

Associated defects:

VSD:	4 (20 %)
PS (Infundibular)	1
PDA:	1
AR:	10 (50 %)
Mild:	2
Moderate:	5
Severe:	3

Agarwal et al (IHJ 1993)

N = 22
Origin

RCC:	14 (63 %)
NCC:	8 (37 %)

Rupture into
  RV: 12
  RA   8

Additional defect:
  VSD: 6 (All associated with RCC origin)
  Perimembranous: 4

  AR: 8
    Severe: 5

Transcatheter closure of ruptured sinus of Valsalva aneurysm using the Amplatzer duct occlude: immediate results and mid-term follow up

P G Kerkar et al
Eur Heart j 2010; 31: 2881-2887

N=   20
Sex: M 12 F 8
Age   17-52 yrs
NYHA Class III / IV   13/20
Exclusion criteria: Co-existing VSD or significant AR requiring
                          surgery
Type of RSOV
  RCC to RA   4
  RCC to RV   5
  outflow
  LCC to RA   10
  LCC to RV inflow   1
Cardiac Catheterization findings
  Defect size   4-11 (Aortic end of defect0
Qp/Qs   1.5 – 3.2
All defect closed from venous side

ADOs used	2-4 mm larger than the aortic side of defect
Success	18/20
Residual shunt	5 (13 had complete closure)
Severity	
Small shunt	4
Moderate	1 (With self abating hemolysis)
Trivial AR	4
Follow up	1-60 months (Median 27 months)
NYHA class I	15
NYHA class II	3

Residual shunt disappeared in 3; small in 2

Procedure related AR vanished in 2 out of 4

No AR progression, recurrence, infective endocarditis or embolization

Conclusion: In appropriately selected cases of ruptured sinus of Valsalva aneurysm, TCC is an attractive alternative to surgery with encouraging short- and mid-term results

Transcatheter device closure of ruptured sinus of Valsalva: not addressing the pathology, does it make a difference

Radhakrishnan et al.

JACC; Vol 62: Issue 18, S1October 2013

N=	13
Age:	39 ± 10.0 yrs
NYHA class	
II	6
III	6
IV:	1

Procedural details

All closed with PDA device
Mean procedural time: 30 ± 5.4 minutes
Mean fluoroscopic time: 20 ± 7 minutes
Hospital stay   2 ± 1.1 days
Mortality   1
Follow up: 1 month – 5 yrs (Mean 3 yrs)
All patients in NTHA class I
All had complete closure of shunt

Conclusion:

Transcatheter closure of isolated RSOV is a viable alternative to surgical repair with good outcome on echocardiographic follow up. Though a long term data is required particularly with respect to aortic root distortion evaluated by other imaging modality like CT scan or MRI.

Abbreviations

AA:	Aortoarteritis
A2C:	Apical two chamber
A4C:	Apical four chamber
A5C:	Apical five chamber
ACR:	American College of Rheumatology
ADO:	Amplatzer Duct Occluder
AF:	Atrial Fibrillation
ALCAPA:	Anomalous origin of left coronary artery from pulmonary artery
ANCA:	Anti-neutrophic cytoplasmic antibody
ANF:	Antinuclear Factor
AP:	Aortopulmonary
AR:	Aortic Regurgitation
AS:	Aortic Stenosis
ASD:	Atrial septal defect
ASO:	Antistreptolysin
ASO:	Amplatzer Septal Occluder
ASOV:	Aneurysm of sinus of Valsalva
ATL:	Anterior tricuspid leaflet
AV:	Atrioventricular
AV:	Arteriovenous
AVR:	Aortiv valve replacement
BP:	Blood pressure
CABG:	Coronary artery bypass graft
CAD:	Coronary artery disease
CCF:	Congestive cardiac failure
CHB:	Complete heart block
CHD:	Congenital heart disease
CHF:	Congestive heart failure
CRP:	C-reactive protein

CT:	Computed tomography
CXR:	Chest X-ray
DCM:	Dilated Cardiomyopathy
D/D:	Differential diagnosis
DSA:	Digital subtraction angiography
ECG:	Electrocardiogram
EDM:	Early diastolic murmur
EF:	Ejection fraction
E/O:	Evidence of
ESM:	Ejection systolic murmur
ESR:	Erythrocyte sedimentation rate
F/U:	Follow up
Fr:	French
GI:	Gastrointestinal
HBP:	High blood pressure
HLA:	Human Leukocyte antigen
HT:	Hypertension
IAS:	Interatrial septum
ICS:	Intercostal space
IE:	Infective endocarditis
IgA:	Immunoglobulin A
IgG:	Immunoglobulin G
IgM:	Immunoglobulin M
IHJ:	Indian Heart Journal
IRBBB:	Incomplete right bundle branch block
IUGR:	Intrauterine growth retardation
IV:	Intra-venous
IVC:	Inferior vena cava
IVS:	Inter ventricular septum
IVUS:	Intravascular Ultrasound
JVP:	Jugular venous pulse
LA:	Left atrium

LAE:	Left atrial enlargement
LAO:	Left anterior oblique
LBBB:	Left bundle branch block
LCC:	Left coronary cusp
LICS:	Left intercostal space
LSB:	Left sterna border
LSCA:	Left subclavian artery
LV:	Left ventricle
LVEF:	Left ventricular ejection fraction
LVF:	Left ventricular failure
LVH:	Left ventricular hypertrophy
LVVO:	Left ventricular volume overload
MPA:	Main pulmonary artery
MR:	Mitral Regurgitation
MDM:	Mid diastolic murmur
MRI:	Magnetic resonance imaging
NCC:	Non coronary cusp
NYHA:	New York Heart Association
P2:	Pulmonary component of second heart sound
PA:	Pulmonary artery
PA:	Postero-anterior
PDA:	Patent ductus arteriosus
PH:	Pulmonary hypertension
PLAX:	Parasternal long axis
PS:	Pulmonary stenosis
PSAX:	Parasternal short axis
PSM:	Pansystolic murmur
PTBA:	Percutaneous Transluminal Balloon Angioplasty
PTFE:	Polytetrafluoroethylene
PV:	Pulmonary valve
RA:	Right atrium
RAE:	Right atrial enlargement
RAO:	Right anterior oblique
RAP:	Right atrial pressure

RBBB:	Right bundle branch block
RCA:	Right coronary artery
RCC:	Right coronary cusp
RSOV:	Ruptured sinus of Valsalva
RV:	Right ventricle
RVH:	Right ventricular hypertrophy
RVOT:	Right ventricle outflow tract
Rx:	Treatment
SM:	Systolic murmur
SOV:	Sinus of Valsalva
STL:	Septal tricuspid leaflet
STS:	Society of Thoracic Surgeons
SV:	Sinus of Valsalva
SVA:	Sinus of Valsalva aneurysm
TA:	Takayasu arteritis
TEE:	Trans esophageal echocardiography
TTE:	Trans thoracic echocardiography
TR:	Tricuspid Regurgitation
TV:	Tricuspid valve
VSD:	Ventricular septal defect
VTI:	Velocity time integral

Suggested Readings

Aortoarteritis

1. Nasu T. Pathology of pulseless disease: A systematic study andcritical review of twenty-one autopsy cases reported in Japan. Angiology. 1963;14:225–242. [PubMed: 13937653]
2. Sen PK, Kinare SG, Kelkar MD, Parulkar GB. Nonspecific Aortoarteritis-A Monographi Based on a Study of 101 cases. Bombay:Tata McGraw-Hill publishing Co; 1972.
3. Lupi-Herrera E, Sanchez-Torres G, Marcushamer J, Mispireta J, Horwitz S, Vela JE. Takayasu's arteritis. Clinical study of 107 cases. Am Heart J. 1977;93:94–103. [PubMed: 12655]
4. Ishikawa K. Natural history and classification of occlusive thromboartopathy (Takayasu's disease) Circulation. 1978; 57:27–35.[PubMed: 21760]
5. Takayasu M. Case with unusual changes of the central vessels in the retina (in Japanese) Acta Soc Ophthal Jap. 1908;12:554–555.
6. Waern AU, Andersson P, Hemmingson A. Takayasu's arteritis: A hospital region based study on occurrence, treatment and prognosis. Angiology. 1983;34:311–320. [PubMed: 6133485]
7. Kinare SG, Gandhi MS, Deshpande JR. Mumbai: 1998. Nonspecific aortoarteritis (pathology and radiology) monograph published by Quest publications.
8. Ishikawa K. Diagnostic approach and proposed criteria for the clinical diagnosis of Takayasu's arteriopathy. J Am Coll Cardiol.1988;12:964–972. [PubMed: 2901440]
9. Arend WP, Michel BA, Bloch DA, Hunder GG, Calobrese lH, Edworthy SM, et al. The American College of Rheumatology

1990 criteria for the classification of Takayasu arteritis. Arthritis Rheumatism. 1990;33:1129–1132. [PubMed: 1975175]

10. Sharma S, Rajani M, Talwar KK. Angiographic morphology in nonspecific aortoarteritis (Takayasu's arteritis): a study of 126 patients from north India. Cardiovasc Intervent Radiol. 1992;15:160–165.[PubMed: 1352736]

11. Tyagi S, Kaul UA, Satsangi DK, Arora R. Percutaneous transluminal angioplasty for renovascular hypertension in children: Initial and long term results. Pediatrics. 1997;99:44–49. [PubMed: 8989336]

12. Sharma S, Saxena A, Talwar KK, Kaul U, Mehta SN, Rajani M. Renal artery stenosis caused by nonspecific arteritis (Takayasu disease): Results of treatment with percutaneous transluminal angioplasty. AJR AM J Roentgenol. 1992;158:417–422. [PubMed:1346073]

13. Talwar KK, Chopra P, Narula JS, Shrivastava S, Singh SK, Sharma S, Saxena A, Rajani M, Bhatia ML. Myocardial involvement and its response to immunosuppressive therapy in non specific aortoarteritis (Takayasu's disease) – A study by endomyocardial biopsy. Int J Cardiol.1988;23:323–334. [PubMed: 2906633]

14. Talwar KK, Kumar K, Chopra P, Sharma S, Shrivastava S, Wasir HS, et al. Cardiac involvement in non-specific aortoarteritis (Takayasu's arteritis) Am Heart J. 1991;122:166–1670.

15. Lee HY, Rao PS. Percutaneous transluminal angioplasty in Takayasu's arteritis. Am Heart J. 1996;132:1084–1086. [PubMed:8892798]

16. Sharma S, Kamalakar T, Rajani M, Talwar KK, Shrivastava S. The incidence and patterns of pulmonary artery involvement in Takayasu's arteritis. Clin Radiol. 1990;42:182–187. [PubMed: 1976468]

17. Lagneau P, Michel JB, Wuong PN. Surgical treatment for Takayasu's disease. Ann Surg. 1987;205:157–166. [PMCID:PMC1492814] [PubMed: 2880571]
18. Tyagi S, Khan M, Kaul UA, Arora R. Percutaneous transluminal angioplasty for stenosis of aorta due to aortoarteritis in children. Paed Cardiol. 1999;29:404–410.
19. Bali HK, Jain S, Jain A, Sharma BK. Precutaneous angioplasty and stent placement in Takayasu arteritis. Int J Cardiol. 1998;66 (Suppl I):S213–217. [PubMed: 9951822]
20. Takagi A, Tada Y, Sato O, Miyata T. Surgical treatment of Takayasu's arteritis: A long term follow up study. J Cardiovasc Surg. 1989;30:553–558. [PubMed: 2570782]
21. Subramanyan R, Joy J, Balakrishnan KG. Natural history of aortoarteritis (Takayasu's disease) Circulation. 1989;80:429–437. [PubMed: 2569946]
22. Sharma BK, Jain S, Suri S, Numano F. Diagnostic criteria for Takayasu arteritis. Int J Cardiol 1996;54(Suppl):S141–7.

Sinus of Valsalva

1. Feldman DN, Roman MJ. Aneurysms of the sinus of valsalva. *Cardiology.* 2006;106:73-81.
2. Sakakibara S, Konno S. Congenital aneurysm of the sinus of valsalva associated with ventricular septal defect. Anatomical aspects. *Am Heart J.* 1968;75:595- 603.
3. Perloff JK. The clinical recognition of congenital heart disease. *Philadelphia:*WB Saunders,
4. Fishbein MC, Obma R, Roberts WC. Unruptured sinus of valsalva aneurysm. *Am J Cardiol.* 1975;35:918.
5. Yilmaz AT, Demirkilic U, Ozal E, Tatar H, Ozturk OY. Aneurysms of the sinus of valsalva. *J Cardiovasc Surg.* 1997;38:119-24.

6. Bonfils-Roberts EA, DuShane JW, McGoon DC, Danielson GK. Aortic sinus fistula-surgical considerations and results of operation. *Annals of Thoracic Surgery.* 1971;12:492-502

7. Sakakibara, S., Konno, S. Congenital aneurysm of the sinus of Valsalva(Anatomy and classification). Am Heart J. 1962;63:405–424.

8. Dong, C., Wu, Q.-Yu, Tang, Y. Ruptured sinus of Valsalva aneurysm(A Beijing experience). Ann Thorac Surg. 2002; 74:1621–1624.

9. Choudhary, S.K., Bhan, A., Sharma, R. et al, Sinus of Valsalva aneurysms(20 years' experience). J Card Surg. 1997;12:300–308.

10. Naka, Y., Kadoba, K., Ohtake, S. et al, The long-term outcome of a surgical repair of sinus of Valsalva aneurysm. Ann Thorac Surg. 2000;70:727–729.

11. Jones, A.M., Langley, F.A. Aortic sinus aneurysms. Br Heart J. 1949;11:325–341.

12. Mohanakrishnan, L., Vijayakumar, K., Sukumaran, P. et al, Unruptured sinus of Valsalva aneurysm with right ventricular outflow obstruction. Asian Cardiovasc Thorac Ann. 2003;11:74–76.

13. Desai, A.G., Sharma, S., Kumar, A. et al, Echocardiographic diagnosis of unruptured aneurysm of right sinus of Valsalva(An unusual cause of right ventricular outflow obstruction). Am Heart J. 1985;109:363–364.

14. Warnes, C.A., Maron, B.J., Jones, M. et al, Asymptomatic sinus of Valsalva aneurysm causing right ventricular outflow obstruction before and after rupture. Am J Cardiol. 1984;54:1383–1384.

15. Dev, V., Goswami, K.C., Shrivastava, S. et al, Echocardiographic diagnosis of aneurysm of the sinus of Valsalva. Am Heart J. 1993;126:930–936.

16. Shah, R.P., Ding, Z.P., Ng, A.S. et al, A ten-year review of ruptured sinus of Valsalva(Clinico-pathological and echo-Doppler features). Singapore Med J. 2001;42:473–476.

17. Ogawa, T., Iwama, Y., Hashimoto, H. et al, Noninvasive methods in the diagnosis of ruptured aneurysm of Valsalva(Usefulness of magnetic resonance imaging and Doppler echocardiography). Chest. 1991;100:579–581.

18. Cheng, T.O. Nonsurgical closure of rupture of aneurysm of sinus of Valsalva. Catheter Cardiovasc Interv. 2003;58:412.

19. Rao, P.S., Bromberg, B.I., Jureidini, S.B. et al, Transcatheter occlusion of ruptured sinus of Valsalva aneurysm(Innovative use of available technology). Catheter Cardiovasc Interv. 2003;58:130–134.

20. McGoon, D.C., Edwards, J.E., Kirklin, J.W. Surgical treatment of ruptured aneurysm of aortic sinus. Ann Surg. 1958;147:387–392.

21. Sakakibara, S., Konno, S. Congenital aneurysm of the sinus of Valsalva(Criteria for recommending surgery). Am J Cardiol. 1963;12:100–106.

22. Cooley, D.A. in: Techniques in Cardiac Surgery. Ed 2. Saunders, Philadelphia, PA; 1984.

23. Cooley, D.A. Surgical Treatment of Aortic Aneurysms. Saunders, Philadelphia, PA; 1986.

About the Author

Dr. Alok Ranjan is a senior interventional cardiologist. He has completed his cardiology training from prestigious G S Seth Medical college and KEM Hospital, Mumbai, India. He has worked as cardiology fellow in Glasgow Royal Infirmary, Glasgow for 1 year. After completion of fellowship he has been practicing cardiology in Gujarat, India for last fifteen years. He has vast experience in Coronary as well as Rheumatic heart disease (RHD). He is co-author of a book called "Patel's Atlas on Transradial Interventions: The basics."Apart from this, he has published five handbooks from AuthorHouse related to Rheumatic Fever and Valvular Heart Diseases. This handbook deals with Aortoarteritis and Ruptured Sinus of Valsalva. This handbook will be a very good reference book for students as well as medical practitioners.

Printed in the United States
By Bookmasters